# Doing Couple Therapy

**THE GUILFORD FAMILY THERAPY SERIES**
Michael P. Nichols, Series Editor

Recent Volumes

Doing Couple Therapy:
Craft and Creativity in Work with Intimate Partners
*Robert Taibbi*

Doing Family Therapy, Second Edition:
Craft and Creativity in Clinical Practice
*Robert Taibbi*

Collaborative Therapy with Multi-Stressed Families, Second Edition
*William C. Madsen*

Working with Families of the Poor, Second Edition
*Patricia Minuchin, Jorge Colapinto, and Salvador Minuchin*

Couple Therapy with Gay Men
*David E. Greenan and Gil Tunnell*

Beyond Technique in Solution-Focused Therapy:
Working with Emotions and the Therapeutic Relationship
*Eve Lipchik*

Emotionally Focused Couple Therapy with Trauma Survivors:
Strengthening Attachment Bonds
*Susan M. Johnson*

# Doing
# Couple
# Therapy

## Craft and Creativity in Work
## with Intimate Partners

### Robert Taibbi

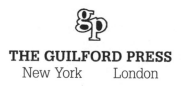

**THE GUILFORD PRESS**
New York    London

*To my family*

*Susan*
*Chris, Joan, and Josh*
*Jenn*
*Gabriel and Freya*
*Stanley and Marion*
*Molly*

© 2009 The Guilford Press
A Division of Guilford Publications, Inc.
72 Spring Street, New York, NY 10012
www.guilford.com

Paperback edition 2011

Printed in the United States of America

This book is printed on acid-free paper.

Last digit is print number:  9  8  7  6  5  4  3

**Library of Congress Cataloging-in-Publication Data**

Taibbi, Robert.
     Doing couple therapy : craft and creativity in work with
intimate partners / Robert Taibbi.
          p. ; cm. — (Guilford family therapy series)
     Includes bibliographical references and index.
     ISBN 978-1-60623-244-6 (hardcover : alk. paper)
     ISBN 978-1-60918-204-5 (paperback : alk. paper)
     1. Couples therapy.   I. Title. II. Series: Guilford family
therapy series.
     [DNLM: 1. Couples Therapy—methods. 2. Marital
Therapy—methods.  WM 430.5.M3 T129d 2009]
     RC488.5.T327 2009
     616.89′1562—dc22
                                                    2009003206